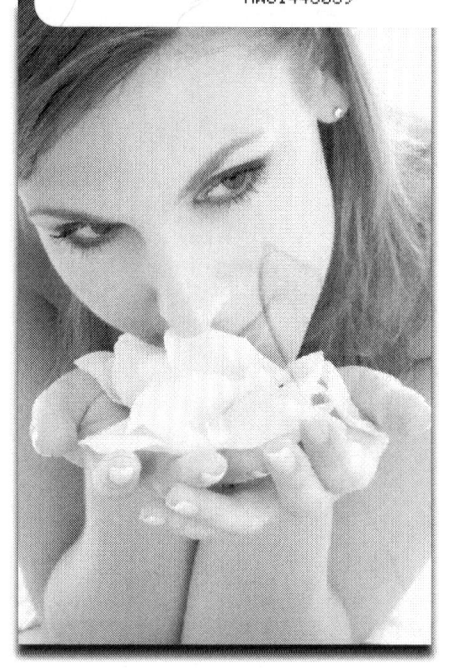

Custom Massage Therapy Oils

A DIY Guide to Therapeutic Recipes for Homemade Massage Oils
(The Art of the Bath Vol. 1)

Alynda Carroll

Ordinary Matters Publishing
P.O. Box 430577
Houston, TX 77243

www.OrdinaryMattersPublishing.com

Custom Massage Therapy Oils
A DIY Guide to Therapeutic Recipes for Homemade Massage Oils

Copyright © 2014 Ordinary Matters Publishing
All rights reserved worldwide

ISBN-13: 978-1-941303-10-8 (paperback)
ISBN-10: 1941303102
First Printing: October, 2014

Cover: Peter Arnott

All rights reserved. No part of this book may be reproduced in any form or by any electronic or mechanical means, including information storage and retrieval systems, without permission in writing from the author, except in the case of brief quotations used in critical articles or reviews. This means that you cannot record or photocopy any material, ideas, or tips that are provided in this book. Requests for permission should be addressed to the publisher.

Disclaimer and Terms of Use: Although the author and publisher have made every effort to ensure that the information in this book was correct at press time, the author and publisher to not assume and hereby disclaim any liability to any party for any loss, damage, or disruption caused by errors or omissions, whether such omissions result from negligence, accident, or any other cause. The author and the publisher do not warrant the accuracy of the information, text, and graphics contained within the book due to the rapidly changing nature of science, research, known and unknown facts, and the Internet. This book is presented solely for informational and entertainment purposes only.

Printed in the United States of America

Books by Alynda Carroll

The Art of the Bath Series

Custom Massage Therapy Oils
A DIY Guide to Therapeutic Recipes for Homemade Massage Oils

A DIY Guide to Therapeutic Bath Enhancements
Homemade Recipes for Bath Salts, Melts, Bombs & Scrubs

A DIY Guide to Therapeutic Body & Skin Care Recipes
Homemade Body Lotions, Skin Creams, Gels, Whipped Butters, Herbal Balms and Salves

A DIY Guide to Therapeutic Spa Treatments
Homemade Recipes for the Face, Hands, Feet & Body

A DIY Guide to Therapeutic Body Butters
A Beginner's Guide to Homemade Body and Hair Butters

A DIY Guide to Therapeutic Natural Hair Care Recipes
A Beginner's Guide to Homemade Shampoos, Conditioners, Rinses, Gels and Sprays

Life Hacks for Everyday Living Series

HOUSEHOLD HACKS
Super Simple Ways to Clean Your Home Effortlessly Using Hydrogen Peroxide and Other Cleaning Secrets

Pick up your FREE report *Learn the Art of Self-Massage*:

http://www.ordinarymatterspublishing.com/massage-bonus

Praise for *The Art of the Bath* series

for *A DIY Guide to Therapeutic Spa Treatments from the Comfort of Your Home*

"Ahhhh this is a keeper! It's packed with awesome and easy to make spa like treatments. I love going to the spa, but in between spa treatments this book is as good as it gets. My favorites so far are the healthy coconut cuticle softener, the tension-relieving eucalyptus food massage oil treatment- so good oh and for a coffee junkie like me, the all-over coffee body scrub priceless! Great DIY spa treatments book."
~ Yvette (Amazon reviewer)

for *A DIY Guide to Therapeutic Bath Enhancements*

". . . easy to follow and very simple too. If you are looking for a book that you can easily follow and make you feel like a pro in no time when it comes to making soaps, bath salts and scrubs, this is the book to have!"
~ LH Thompson (Amazon reviewer)

for *Custom Massage Therapy Oils*

As well as being relaxing, the benefits of massage can be physical as well as mental. This book is a great little guide to their therapeutic benefits, how to make your own massage oil and which blends are recommended to induce sleep, invigorate or enliven, boost the immune system and more. I will be taking the advice in this book on board, as I know how wonderful massage oils can be - it's just a case of knowing which ones are right to use, depending on the mood and/or benefits you want to induce in the person receiving the massage." ~ Anna J (Amazon reviewer)

for *The Art of the Bath series*

"I love Carroll's DIY Bath series. They are all so welcoming and are full of all these great ideas. Must have." ~ Laura Pope (Amazon reviewer)

"An oil massage, a hot bath, a good night's sleep, soft smells and music, and clothes with soft texture denote sensuality to me."

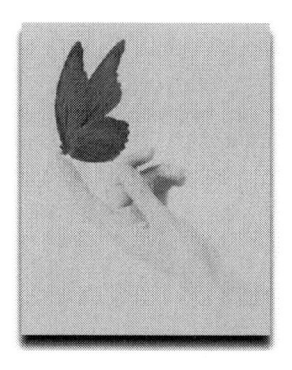

~ Padma Lakshmi

A Note to the Reader

Have you ever had a massage? Remember how wonderful it felt? Left you relaxed, calm, and stress-free. Perhaps it's that relaxation and calmness that you equate with a massage. Maybe, like me, you even add some reduction of pain due to the muscle stretching and relaxing you received. Massages can be helpful in a number of other areas, too.

Most of the time people encounter their first massage due to pain. Their muscles are tight, their backs are in spasm. Their necks hurt. They go because they want relief. Most think you have to make an appointment and go to a massage therapist in order to get that help. Not so. With a bit of creativity, a few good therapy massage oils, and a friend who's willing to help out, you can not only relieve that pain but tackle some other issues as well. (Don't have that extra set of hands around, don't worry. Pick up the special free report on how to *Learn the Art of Self-Massage* offered earlier.)

You might not realize it, but you can easily create your own homemade massage oils to help you sleep. Another combination of therapy oils can increase your immune system, while still another can lower your blood pressure. Within these pages you'll find various massage oil blends that have provided much relief to many who gave them a try. With a dash of creativity, who knows what other ailments you can relieve.

As with anything, you'll want to read up on the essential oils and do the preliminary tests to make sure you don't have any allergies or potential adverse reactions.

Finally, nothing in this book should be construed as an attempt to offer or render a medical opinion or otherwise engage in the practice of medicine. The suggested uses of these oils comes from a wellspring of common knowledge and from some studies and is presented solely for informational and entertainment purposes only.

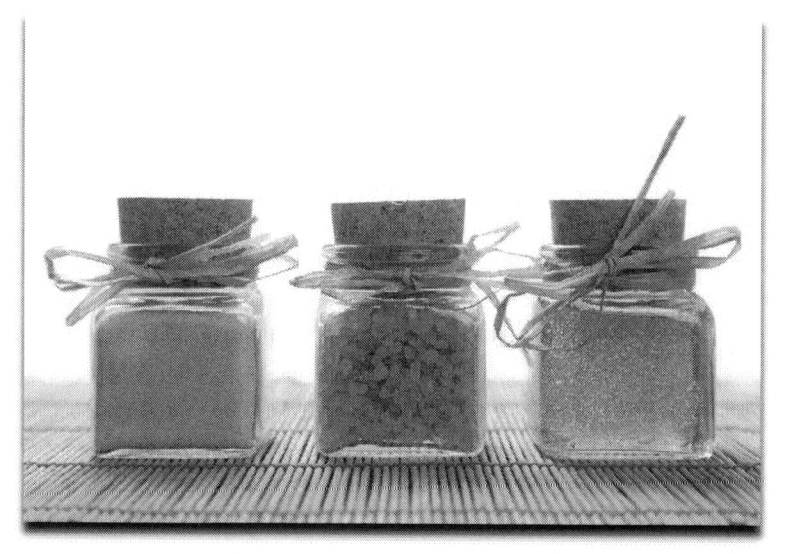

How to Give Yourself a Massage

Thank you for buying this book. In appreciation, I'm offering you this free report:

Learn the Art of Self-Massage

http://www.ordinarymatterspublishing.com/massage-bonus/

CONTENTS

BOOKS BY ALYNDA CARROLL III
A NOTE TO THE READER I
HOW TO GIVE YOURSELF A MASSAGE III
CONTENTS V
INTRODUCTION 1
    SAFETY FIRST! 4
GETTING STARTED 9
SLEEP-INDUCING BLENDS 13
    LAVENDER-CHAMOMILE MASSAGE OIL 15
    NEROLI MASSAGE OIL 16
    SANDALWOOD-CEDARWOOD MASSAGE OIL 17
STRESS REDUCTION BLENDS 19
    SUNFLOWER-GERANIUM MASSAGE OIL 21
    TROPICAL MASSAGE OIL 22
    YLANG YLANG MASSAGE OIL 23
SORE MUSCLE RELIEF BLENDS 25
    MARJORAM-ROMAN-CHAMOMILE MASSAGE OIL 27
    BASIL-JUNIPER-LEMONGRASS MASSAGE OIL 28
    EUCALYPTUS MASSAGE OIL 29
ACHES, PAINS AND RHEUMATISM RELIEF BLENDS 31
    VETIVER MASSAGE OIL 33
    WINTERGREEN-MARJORAM MASSAGE OIL 34
    PEPPERMINT-CHAMOMILE MASSAGE OIL 35
INVIGORATING AND ENLIVENING BLENDS 37

ANISE-ORANGE MASSAGE OIL	39
ROSEMARY-THYME MASSAGE OIL	40
TEA TREE-CYPRESS MASSAGE OIL	41
IMMUNE-BOOSTING BLENDS	**43**
FRANKINCENSE-BERGAMOT MASSAGE OIL	45
HYSSOP-CLARY-SAGE MASSAGE OIL	46
MOUNTAIN SAVORY MASSAGE OIL	47
CONCLUSION	**49**
ABOUT THE AUTHOR	**51**
MORE BOOKS BY ALYNDA CARROLL	53
WHAT'S NEW?	**55**
EXCERPT FROM HOUSEHOLD HACKS	**57**
NOTES	**61**
INDEX	**65**

INTRODUCTION

"You can't turn back the clock but you can wind it up again..." —Bonnie Prudden

What are Massage Oils?

Massage oils are used to moisturize the skin and create a smooth surface, free of friction, in which to perform a massage. Oils derived from plants are the most popular "base" or "carrier" oils. These oils contain vitamins and nutrients which are beneficial when used alone. When the essential oils of aromatic herbs, flowers and plants are combined with these base oils, the benefits of the massage and the overall massage experience are heightened.

What are Custom Therapeutic Massage Oils?

The list of essential oils that can be used to enhance massage therapy is long and growing longer as the known healing properties of plants continues to be studied. Since many plants have similar therapeutic qualities, it is possible to create custom blends based on aromas that are the most pleasing to each person, while gaining the same benefits. One essential oil can address both emotional and physical issues, so the addition of just one of these oils to the base oil will deliver therapeutic and non-therapeutic benefits.

Therapeutic Benefits of Massage Oils

- Improves circulation
- Soothes aches and pains
- Relieves cramping muscles and muscle spasms
- Detoxifies
- Drains the lymphatic system
- Aids in joint flexibility
- Reduces anxiety and nervous tension
- Encourages deep sleep
- Regulates cardio and respiratory rhythms
- Lowers blood pressure
- Boosts the immune system

Non-Therapeutic Benefits of Massage Oils

- Aids in meditation
- Uplifts the spirit
- Promotes cheerfulness
- Helps restore spiritual energy and balance
- Stimulates the mood

- Improves energy

Although massage oils with added essential oils are readily available for purchase, it is easy, cheaper, and way more fun to customize your own special blends at home. Besides creating blends to meet personal needs, homemade massage oils make great gifts for friends and family.

There are many oils that can be used as "base" or "carrier" oil to dilute the ultra-concentrated essential oils. It is not advised to use essential oils alone on the skin, since they can cause irritation or an allergic reaction. The recipes in this book use five of the most readily available, least reactive, basic oils. These oils also provide additional vitamins, proteins and minerals.

5 Basic Carrier Oils

There are five common carrier oils that are found to be the best to use when mixing massage oils.

Sweet Almond Oil –Rich in fatty acids, this oil soothes, softens and reconditions the skin.

Apricot Kernel Oil – This oil works great for all skin types, but is especially beneficial to sensitive or aged skin.

Jojoba Oil – This oil is known for its advanced molecular stability, making it most like the skin's own sebum. Because of this, it absorbs rapidly and smoothly into the skin during a massage.

Fractionated Coconut Oil – This odorless oil moisturizes the skin while adding a protective layer, making it quite beneficial for sensitive skin or skin that is irritated or inflamed.

Sunflower Oil – High in Vitamins A, D, E and Oleic and unsaturated fatty acids, this oil is a good choice for very dry or damaged skin.

SAFETY FIRST!

Essential oils are highly concentrated components of certain plants and should be treated with special care. Whenever creating massage oils at home, it's important to keep these things in mind:

- Never use essential oils directly on the skin. Always dilute with carrier oils before using.

- Keep all essential oils out of the reach of children.

- Never ingest essential oils.

- Always do a skin test before using any essential oil. Do this by dabbing a small amount of oil on the inside of the wrist and cover it with an adhesive bandage for eight hours. After removing the bandage, if there is any sign of irritation, try another one for better results.

- Always consult a physician before using essential oils on the skin if you are pregnant or suffering from a medical condition.

- Some oils are photosensitive, meaning they react to sunlight on the skin. If using these oils, such as citrus or Bergamot, wait 6 hours after using before being in direct sunlight or tanning beds.

- Always dilute essential oils with oil, not water.

- Avoid contact of essential oils with the eyes, nose, mouth, ears or other openings in the body.

- If your eyes come into contact with essential oils, flush them with milk or vegetable oil. Contact a physician, if experiencing irritation.

- Avoid the use of essential oils on pets.

- Don't leaving a bottle or vial of essential oil on wooden surfaces, as it may result in marks or rings.

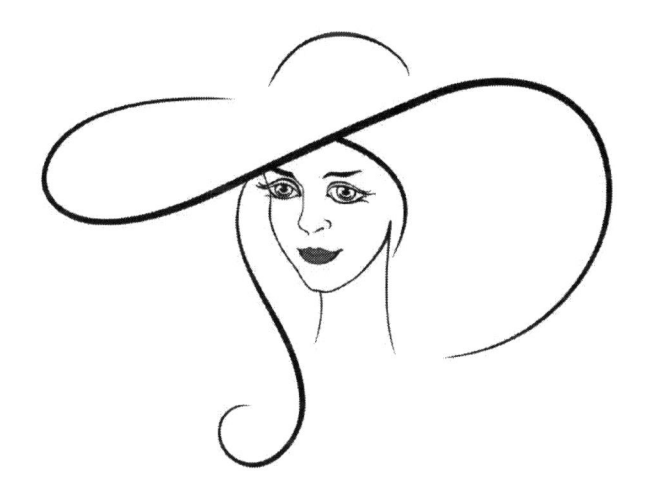

Getting Started

It's easy and affordable to start creating your own special massage oils. Here's what you'll need:

- Your choice of carrier oil

- Essential oils that are pleasing to you and/or are for a specific purpose

- Any dark-colored glass (amber or green) bottle, vial, or jar with cap or lid to protect the oil's potency against deteriorating light.

5 Steps to Making Massage Oil
Take the following preliminary steps to create your own massage oil blend.

1. Choose a carrier oil based on your skin type and the results you want to achieve.

2. Research the various essential oils and choose ones based on your fragrance preference and the healing qualities you desire. Your massage oil may contain as many essential oils as you prefer. All you need to do is mix a little bit of your blend together beforehand to test it, since the fragrance will remain with you for a while after the massage.

3. Add carrier oil to your container first. Then add the essential oils one drop at a time, using a dropper. You may wish to add one drop, mix, and smell before adding another drop, to ensure you don't make your oil too weak or too strong. Mix the ingredients by shaking them well. (Approximately 4 teaspoons of oil are used in a full body massage.)

4. Label each bottle of massage oil, including the name of the carrier oil, the essential oil, the dilution percent, and the date it was mixed.

5. Store your massage oil in the refrigerator.

Dilution Percentages

Use this guide when deciding how much essential oil to dilute in the base oil.

1. Normal Skin - 2 1/2%. For every 4 tsp (20 ml, about 2/3 fl. oz.) of carrier oil, use up to 10 drops of essential oil.

2. Sensitive Skin Dilution - 1%. For every 4 tsp of carrier oil, use up to 5 drops of essential oil.

3. Extra sensitive skin – ½%. For every 4 tsp of carrier oil, use up to 2 drops of essential oil.

You should definitely read up on these and other oils to make sure you know whether it is appropriate oil for you and your needs.

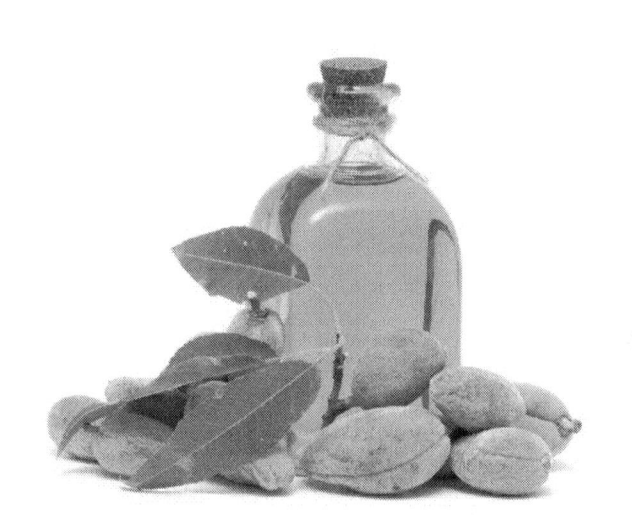

SLEEP-INDUCING BLENDS

LAVENDER-CHAMOMILE MASSAGE OIL

The scent of lavender encourages "slow wave" sleep, or the segment of the sleep cycle when the heart beats slower and the muscles relax. German chamomile creates a calming, sedative effect. Combining the two ensures a good night's rest.

Ingredients:
4 tsp. Jojoba oil
3 drops Lavender essential oil
3 drops German Chamomile essential oil

Directions:

Pour Jojoba oil into a dark glass bottle or container. For every 4 teaspoons of Jojoba oil, add 3 drops of Lavender essential oil, and 3 drops of German Chamomile. Mix well and apply.

NEROLI MASSAGE OIL

Of all the essential oils, Neroli has the strongest sedative properties. This oil is known to ease anxiety and calm fears to allow the best chance of relaxing into a restorative sleep.

Ingredients:
4 tsp. Apricot Kernel oil
8 drops Neroli essential oil

Directions:

In a dark bottle or container, pour the Apricot oil. With a dropper, add 8 drops of Neroli essential oil. Mix well and massage into body.

SANDALWOOD-CEDARWOOD MASSAGE OIL

The essential oil of the exhausted, Sandalwood creates a feeling of calm and deep relaxation, while Cedarwood relieves stress and helps relieve nervous tension to facilitate a deep night's sleep.

Ingredients:
4 tsp. Sweet Almond oil
5 drops Sandalwood essential oil

Directions:

Using a dropper, add 5 drops of Sandalwood essential oil to every 4 teaspoons of Sweet Almond oil in a dark bottle or container. Mix well and apply.

STRESS REDUCTION BLENDS

SUNFLOWER-GERANIUM MASSAGE OIL

The essential oil of geranium has unique properties which can calm the nerves while balancing the adrenal glands to reduce stress.

Ingredients:
4 tsp. Sunflower oil
4 drops Geranium essential oil

Directions:

Pour the base oil and sunflower oil into a dark bottle or container. Add 4 drops of Geranium essential oil. Mix well and massage into body.

TROPICAL MASSAGE OIL

Combining the hydrating effects of coconut oil with the restorative qualities of tangerine essential oil creates a tropical-inspired getaway to calm nervous tension.

Ingredients:
4 tsp. Fractionated Coconut oil
5 drops Tangerine essential oil

Directions:

Combine the Coconut oil with the essential oil of Tangerine in a dark bottle or container, using 5 drops of Tangerine oil for every 4 teaspoons of Coconut oil. Mix well and apply.

YLANG MASSAGE OIL

With the addition of Ylang Ylang essential oil to the soothing qualities of Jojoba, this massage oil can regulate the rhythms of the heart and lungs while calming frayed nerves.

Ingredients:
4 tsp. Jojoba oil
6 drops Ylang Ylang essential oil

Directions:

In a dark bottle or jar, pour in the Jojoba oil. For every 4 teaspoons of Jojoba oil, add 6 drops of Ylang Ylang essential oil. Mix well and massage into body.

SORE MUSCLE RELIEF BLENDS

MARJORAM-ROMAN-CHAMOMILE MASSAGE OIL

This massage oil combines the anti-inflammatory properties of chamomile with the muscle relaxing qualities of marjoram to create a soothing, slightly warming, way to relieve sore muscles.

Ingredients:
4 tsp. Apricot Kernel oil
4 drops Roman Chamomile essential oil
4 drops Marjoram essential oil

Directions:

For every 4 teaspoons of Apricot Kernel oil, add 4 drops of Roman Chamomile essential oil and Marjoram essential oil. Mix well in a dark bottle or container and massage into sore muscles.

BASIL-JUNIPER-LEMONGRASS MASSAGE OIL

There are many kinds of Basil essential oils, but the oil from the genus and species Ocimum basilcum CT methyl chavicol is known as the "natural muscle relaxer." When combined with the anti-spasmodic qualities of Juniper essential oil and Lemongrass essential oil, which have the ability to help repair tendons and ligaments, an effective relief for sore and aching muscles is created.

Ingredients:
4 tsp. Sunflower oil
2 drops Basil essential oil (Ocimum basilcum CT methyl chavicol)
2 drops Juniper essential oil
2 drops Lemongrass essential oil

Directions:

In a dark container or bottle, pour in Sunflower oil. For every 4 teaspoons of oil, add 2 drops of each essential oil. Mix well and massage directly onto cramping, aching, or sore muscles.

EUCALYPTUS MASSAGE OIL

Eucalyptus globulus is the genus and species of the Eucalyptus plant that is most beneficial for sore muscles. It's essential oil contains anti-inflammatory properties, and when mixed with Sweet Almond oil, not only soothes muscle cramps and aches, but also adds beneficial Vitamin E to the skin.

Ingredients:
4 tsp. Sweet Almond oil
3 drops Eucalyptus (Eucalyptus globulus) essential oil

Directions:

Combine 4 teaspoons of Sweet Almond oil to 3 drops of Eucalyptus essential oil in a dark bottle or container. To increase the amount, use 3 drops of essential oil to every 4 teaspoons of base oil. Mix well and apply generously to affected muscles

ACHES, PAINS AND RHEUMATISM RELIEF BLENDS

ALYNDA CARROLL

VETIVER MASSAGE OIL

The root of the vetiver plant creates an essential oil rich in healing qualities, including anti-spasmodic and warming properties, which make it especially effective for rheumatism, sprains, and the pain of arthritis.

Ingredients:
4 tsp. Fractionated Coconut oil
1 drop, to begin with, Vetiver essential oil

Directions:

In a dark container, pour in the coconut oil. Since Vetiver essential oil has a strong odor, it is best to begin with 1 drop of Vetiver essential oil and add more to adjust to your personal preference. Mix well and massage directly onto affected areas.

WINTERGREEN-MARJORAM MASSAGE OIL

Wintergreen essential oil creates a beneficial warming touch. Containing methyl salicylate, it can achieve a cortisone-like result, reducing pain and inflammation from joints and muscles. This massage oil combines Wintergreen with the natural muscle relaxation properties of Marjoram for maximum relief from aches, pain, and rheumatism.

Ingredients:
4 tsp. Sunflower oil
2 drops Wintergreen essential oil
2 drops Marjoram essential oil

Directions:

Pour Sunflower oil into a dark bottle or container. Add 2 drops of Wintergreen essential oil and 2 drops Marjoram essential oil and mix well. Massage into aching joints.

PEPPERMINT-CHAMOMILE MASSAGE OIL

Adding a cooling touch to inflamed areas can speed healing and reduce swelling. Peppermint essential oil has cooling qualities as well as the ability to block pain. When combined with the anti-inflammatory properties of German Chamomile, it becomes an effective way to reduce the aches and pains of arthritis and rheumatism.

Ingredients:
4 tsp. Jojoba oil
2 drops Peppermint essential oil
2 drops German Chamomile oil

Directions:

In a dark bottle or vial, pour in Jojoba oil. Add 2 drops Peppermint essential oil and 2 drops German Chamomile essential oil. Mix well and massage into aching areas.

INVIGORATING AND ENLIVENING BLENDS

ANISE-ORANGE MASSAGE OIL

Combining the licorice spiciness of Anise essential oil with the sweet, fresh citrus fragrance of Orange essential oil, creates an uplifting and invigorating blend to comfort and cheer up the soul.

Ingredients:
4 tsp Sweet Almond Oil
2 drops Anise essential oil
2 drops Orange essential oil

Directions:

In a dark bottle or container, pour 4 teaspoons of Sweet Almond oil. Add in 2 drops of Anise essential oil and 2 drops of orange essential oil. Mix well and apply.

ROSEMARY-THYME MASSAGE OIL

What could be more uplifting than the camphor-acetous smell of Rosemary mixed with the pleasant aroma of Thyme? Both have the ability to conjure feelings of the warmth and security of home and hearth.

Ingredients:
4 tsp. Jojoba oil
2 drops Rosemary essential oil
2 drops Thyme essential oil

Directions:

Add 2 drops of Rosemary essential oil and 2 drops of Thyme essential oil to 4 teaspoons of Jojoba oil in a dark container. Mix well and massage directly onto skin.

TEA TREE-CYPRESS MASSAGE OIL

Tea Tree essential oil has been known for ages as the aroma of renewal. When combined with the piney overtones of Cypress, it creates a massage oil that both centers and enlivens the mind and body.

Ingredients:
4 tsp. Apricot Kernel oil
2 drops Tea Tree essential oil
2 drops Cypress essential oil

Directions:

Pour Apricot Kernel oil into dark bottle or vial. Add 2 drops of Tea Tree essential oil and 2 drops of Cypress essential oil. Mix well and massage into skin.

IMMUNE-BOOSTING BLENDS

FRANKINCENSE-BERGAMOT MASSAGE OIL

Frankincense is thought to be the strongest essential oil for boosting the immune system. It has strong antiseptic qualities, and when combined with the antibiotic properties of Bergamot, it creates a strong defense from germ and bacterial invasions of the immune system.

Ingredients:
4 tsp. Fractionated Coconut oil
2 drops Frankincense essential oil
2 drops Bergamot essential oil

Directions:

In a dark container or bottle, pour in Coconut oil. Add 2 drops of Frankincense essential oil, and 2 drops of Bergamot essential oil. Mix well and massage into throat, chest, back and neck.

HYSSOP-CLARY-SAGE MASSAGE OIL

The ability to eliminate toxins from the body makes Hyssop essential oil a powerful immune system booster. Added to Clary Sage, a natural antibacterial, it creates massage oil uniquely able to support the immune system.

Ingredients:
4 tsp. Apricot Kernel oil
2 drops Hyssop essential oil
2 drops Clary Sage essential oil

Directions:

In a dark bottle or container, pour 4 teaspoons of Apricot Kernel oil. Add to this 2 drops of Hyssop essential oil, and 2 drops of Clary Sage essential oil. Mix well and massage into body, especially the throat, chest, and neck.

MOUNTAIN SAVORY MASSAGE OIL

The genus species Satureja montana of Mountain Savory creates an essential oil with strong immune booster qualities containing anti-infectious, anti-inflammatory, antifungal, anti-parasitic, antibacterial, and antiviral properties as well as stimulating the immune system.

Ingredients:
4 tsp. Sunflower oil
5 drops Mountain Savory essential oil

Directions:

Combine 4 teaspoons of Sunflower oil with 5 drops of Mountain Savory essential oil in a dark bottle or vial. Massage directly onto skin.

Conclusion

Well, what do you think? Are you ready to tackle a homemade custom oil recipe? I want to thank you for your purchase of this guide to make massage oils with essential oils right in your very own home. I hope that you've learned something new, and perhaps even have begun to experiment with these different blends.

Over time, you'll be able to perfect your mixing method, and know the power of a variety of different essential oils. You can also expand your collection of different essential oil bottles, as each blend only uses a few drops. A bottle of oil can go a long way.

The possibilities are limited by your creativity. I wish you the best with your health endeavors, and hope that these recipes can get you started on the path to relieve any health problems or stressors you are experiencing. Thank you again and enjoy!

Alynda Carroll

PS: I hope you've enjoyed this book and will take a few minutes to leave a review. Reviews are a big help for authors as well as readers.

ALYNDA CARROLL

About the Author

Alynda Carroll has loved baths since she was a little girl. Bubble baths, lotions, and creams have fascinated her. She spent many hours watching her mom create homemade beauty recipes. Later, Alynda's interests expanded to include herbs, essential oils, aromatherapy and the art of the bath as it is today.

Be sure and buy the rest of Alynda Carroll's best-selling books that make up her popular series The Art of the Bath, s well as her new series Life Hacks for Everyday Living. Look for the excerpt from her new book HOUSEHOLD HACKS at the back of this book.

MORE BOOKS BY ALYNDA CARROLL

The Art of the Bath Series

Custom Massage Therapy Oils: A DIY Guide to Therapeutic Recipes for Homemade Massage Oils

A DIY Guide to Therapeutic Bath Enhancements: Homemade Recipes for Bath Salts, Melts, Bombs & Scrubs

A DIY Guide to Therapeutic Body & Skin Care Recipes: Homemade Body Lotions, Skin Creams, Gels, Whipped Butters, Herbal Balms & Salves

A DIY Guide to Therapeutic Spa Treatments: Homemade Recipes for the Face, Hands, Feet & Body

A DIY Guide to Therapeutic Body Butters: A Beginner's Guide to Homemade Body and Hair Butters

A DIY Guide to Therapeutic Natural Hair Care Recipes: A Beginner's Guide to Homemade Shampoos, Conditioners, Rinses, Gels and Sprays

Life Hacks for Everyday Living *(New Series)*

HOUSEHOLD HACKS: Super Simple Ways to Clean Your Home Effortlessly Using Hydrogen Peroxide and Other Cleaning Secrets

ALYNDA CARROLL

What's New?

Turn the page to read an excerpt from HOUSEHOLD HACKS. To receive updates on the release of Alynda Carroll's next books in the Art of the Bath series and BEAUTY HACKS, go to:

www.SimpleLivingHacks.com

Excerpt from
HOUSEHOLD HACKS

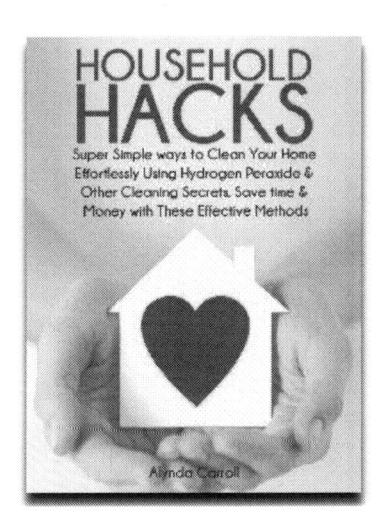

Welcome to Household Hacks, my personal collection of more than 200 cleaning tips, tricks, and household hacks for all areas of the home with an emphasis on using natural, inexpensive cleaners and strategies. Many have been around for a long time, but others are focused on the way we live today.

The advantages are many. You'll save money, time, and energy. You'll also become more effective at housecleaning by using these tips and strategies that will free up your time.

You'll find information about well-seasoned natural cleaners that have been helping people clean for generations and understand why they are gaining popularity today.

You'll discover cleaning strategies and hacks for various rooms including the kitchen, bathroom, and bedroom, as well as the home office. You'll even find creative living hacks to make home life easier.

This collection captures my favorites and includes additional hints and alternatives. If you already have a deep interest in DIY household hacks and natural cleaners, you will probably come across some familiar cleaning remedies. They will serve as reminders, but be of more interest to readers who are just starting down this more natural and simplified way of living. However, newer strategies and ideas will encourage you on your own journey toward living a more natural, clean, and simple life.

A major plus about having this book is that everything is gathered in this one place. This is a good, fun, and definitely useful reference to have on hand.

How the Book is Organized

The book begins by taking a look at the top natural cleaners in use today. There are several cleaning hacks and tips for each cleaner. I like to have a list of things I can do with a particular cleaner, as well as a collection of cleaning tips particular to an area of the home. The second section offers additional cleaning suggestions and creative household hacks for the kitchen, bathroom, bedroom, laundry and closet, living room, home office, and, by extension, the car.

- ❑ Natural Cleaners
- ❑ Hydrogen Peroxide
- ❑ Vinegar
- ❑ Baking Soda
- ❑ Lemon and lemon juice
- ❑ Apple Cider Vinegar
- ❑ Salt
- ❑ Household Hacks
- ❑ Office and Technology
- ❑ Bathroom
- ❑ Kitchen
- ❑ Bedroom
- ❑ Laundry and Closet
- ❑ Car
- ❑ Creative Hacks

Now that you have an idea of what *HOUSEHOLD HACKS* contains, are you ready to discover its treasures?

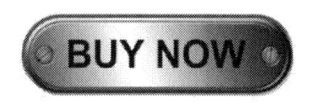

BUY NOW

Buy your copy of *HOUSEHOLD HACKS* today.
www.SimpleLivingHacks.com

ALYNDA CARROLL

NOTES

#ALYNDA CARROLL

CUSTOM MASSAGE THERAPY OILS

ALYNDA CARROLL

INDEX

BOOKS BY ALYNDA CARROLL III
A NOTE TO THE READER I
HOW TO GIVE YOURSELF A MASSAGE III
CONTENTS V
INTRODUCTION 1
   What are Massage Oils? 1
   What are Custom Therapeutic Massage Oils? 1
   Therapeutic Benefits of Massage Oils 2
   Non-Therapeutic Benefits of Massage Oils 2
   5 Basic Carrier Oils 3
   SAFETY FIRST! 4
GETTING STARTED 9
   5 Steps to Making Massage Oil 9
   Dilution Percentages 10
SLEEP-INDUCING BLENDS 13
   LAVENDER-CHAMOMILE MASSAGE OIL 15
   NEROLI MASSAGE OIL 16
   SANDALWOOD-CEDARWOOD MASSAGE OIL 17
STRESS REDUCTION BLENDS 19
   SUNFLOWER-GERANIUM MASSAGE OIL 21
   TROPICAL MASSAGE OIL 22
   YLANG YLANG MASSAGE OIL 23
SORE MUSCLE RELIEF BLENDS 25
   MARJORAM-ROMAN-CHAMOMILE MASSAGE OIL 27

BASIL-JUNIPER-LEMONGRASS MASSAGE OIL 28
　　EUCALYPTUS MASSAGE OIL 29
ACHES, PAINS AND RHEUMATISM RELIEF BLENDS **31**
　　VETIVER MASSAGE OIL 33
　　WINTERGREEN-MARJORAM MASSAGE OIL 34
　　PEPPERMINT-CHAMOMILE MASSAGE OIL 35
INVIGORATING AND ENLIVENING BLENDS **37**
　　ANISE-ORANGE MASSAGE OIL 39
　　ROSEMARY-THYME MASSAGE OIL 40
　　TEA TREE-CYPRESS MASSAGE OIL 41
IMMUNE-BOOSTING BLENDS **43**
　　FRANKINCENSE-BERGAMOT MASSAGE OIL 45
　　HYSSOP-CLARY-SAGE MASSAGE OIL 46
　　MOUNTAIN SAVORY MASSAGE OIL 47
CONCLUSION **49**
ABOUT THE AUTHOR **51**
　　MORE BOOKS BY ALYNDA CARROLL 53
　　　The Art of the Bath Series *53*
　　　Life Hacks for Everyday Living (New Series) *53*
WHAT'S NEW? **55**
EXCERPT FROM HOUSEHOLD HACKS **57**
NOTES **61**
INDEX **65**

Made in the USA
Middletown, DE
02 July 2023